Simone Nantes de Souza

Peritoneal Balance Test

Simone Nantes de Souza

Peritoneal Balance Test

The role of the professional nurse

ScienciaScripts

Imprint

Any brand names and product names mentioned in this book are subject to trademark, brand or patent protection and are trademarks or registered trademarks of their respective holders. The use of brand names, product names, common names, trade names, product descriptions etc. even without a particular marking in this work is in no way to be construed to mean that such names may be regarded as unrestricted in respect of trademark and brand protection legislation and could thus be used by anyone.

Cover image: www.ingimage.com

This book is a translation from the original published under ISBN 978-613-9-69894-3.

Publisher:
Sciencia Scripts
is a trademark of
Dodo Books Indian Ocean Ltd. and OmniScriptum S.R.L publishing group

120 High Road, East Finchley, London, N2 9ED, United Kingdom
Str. Armeneasca 28/1, office 1, Chisinau MD-2012, Republic of Moldova, Europe
Printed at: see last page
ISBN: 978-620-8-14254-4

Summary

Introduction

The general objective of this study was to describe the PET - Peritoneal Equilibrium Test, focusing on the role of nurses in carrying it out, through specific objectives such as defining renal replacement therapies, establishing the role of nursing in peritoneal dialysis and the objectives of the Peritoneal Membrane Test - PET, and finally, describing the role of nursing and the nursing team in carrying out the PET.

The methodology used to construct this work was based on summarising studies on the subject through a vast search of bibliographic references. The main sources consulted for the bibliographical review were articles in scientific journals, books, theses, dissertations and conference abstracts.

Searches were carried out in five bibliographic databases - PubMed, Web of Science, Scielo, Cumulative Index to Nursing and Allied Health Literature (CINAHL) and LILACS - and articles published between 2007 and 2017 were selected. Due to the vast terminology surrounding the subject, we opted to search for free terms, without using controlled vocabulary (descriptors).

When we talk about vital organs, we immediately think of the heart, but is this the only organ that provides life? If we stop to think about it, we'll realise that each system has its function in our body and that these together make up our vital functions.

Physiological elimination is vital for humans. We need to eliminate toxins, minerals and everything that is in excess in our bodies, and this requires a balance between what we ingest (water and food) and eliminate (sweat, urine and faeces).

When it comes to physiological elimination, we have renal elimination, where all the blood volume **passes through the kidneys to be "filtered". The** basic **work of the kidneys** is to produce urine.

Renal failure can be acute or chronic, see the main characteristics of each in table 01 below:

Acute renal failure - ARF	Chronic renal failure - CRF
Rapid loss of kidney function that can be recovered within a few weeks. Causes include dehydration, poisoning, trauma, medication and some diseases. Depending on the severity and because life is not possible without functioning kidneys, dialysis may be necessary.	Slowly progressive, irreversible loss of kidney function (it is at this stage that patients are advised to begin a personal journey of preparation for dialysis).

Table 01-   Source: Dialysis Portal   -2016
https://www.portaldadialise.com/portal/insuficiencia-renal

Dialysis replaces renal function in the removal of toxins, the balance of fluids and electrolytes and the acid-base balance through the process of diffusion and convection. It is known that each chronic renal patient can undergo this renal replacement therapy through haemodialysis, peritoneal dialysis or renal transplantation (TEIXEIRA, 2011).

Peritoneal dialysis, the focus of our study, is a blood purification process in which the transfer of solutes and liquids occurs through a semi-permeable membrane (the peritoneum) that separates two compartments. One is the abdominal cavity, where the dialysis solution is contained; the other is the peritoneal capillary, where blood containing excess nitrogenous slags, potassium and other substances is found. The peritoneum acts as a filter, allowing mass transfer between the two compartments. It consists of a semi-permeable, heterogeneous membrane with multiple pores of different sizes (BLAKE ET.AL, 2003).

Each patient has unique characteristics when it comes to transport through the peritoneal membrane, and these characteristics can be assessed using the mass transfer area coefficient (MTAC), standard permeability analysis and the peritoneal equilibrium test (PET), which is the focus of this study.

Patients on peritoneal dialysis undergo the peritoneal equilibrium test (PET) to assess the rate of transfer of solutes and water across the peritoneal membrane. This test is based on three parameters: ratio of creatinine in the dialysate to plasma at 4 hours (Creatinine D/P); ratio of glucose in the dialysate at 4 and 0 hours (glucose D/D0); ultrafiltration volume at 4 hours (UFV). This research is necessary with a focus on the process of assessing peritoneal balance and the need for a multi-professional team to assess, carry out and apply peritoneal dialysis (ROMÃO JUNIOR, 2004).

Renal replacement therapy by peritoneal dialysis can be carried out according to Ordinance No. 389 of 13 March 2014 by:
Continuous ambulatory peritoneal dialysis (CAPD);
Automatic peritoneal dialysis (APD);
Intermittent peritoneal dialysis (IPD).

In this context, we see nursing as a key factor in the process of orientating, choosing and carrying out PD. PET scans are essential for carrying out this therapy, as they allow patients to be classified according to the solute transport characteristics of the peritoneal membrane, as well as assessing ultrafiltration characteristics. The PET scan requires detailed supervision, especially by the nursing team.

CHAPTER 1

Anatomy and physiology of the kidneys

The sciences of anatomy and physiology are the foundation for understanding the structures and functions of the human body. Anatomy is the science of structure and its relationships. For AIRES (2008, p. 5), physiology is the science of the body's functions, i.e. how the body's parts work. As function is never completely separate from structure, we understand the human body better by studying physiology and anatomy together. Each structure of the body is designed to fulfil a specific function and how a part is structured often determines the functions it can perform.

Anatomy is the science that aims to show in great detail the shape and location of each organ, identifying its potential and analysing the structure of each part of the body (TORTORA, DERRICKSON, 2017, p.9).

1. Anatomy

To begin our study, it is important to consider the importance of the organs and systems that make up the urinary system, so let's recall the general anatomy and physiology of the urinary system, so that we can understand renal insufficiency and consequently renal replacement therapies.

1.1 - Anatomical Skeletal Positions

By using unified terms, we have the various anatomical positions. The standard position is called the anatomical description position or anatomical position.

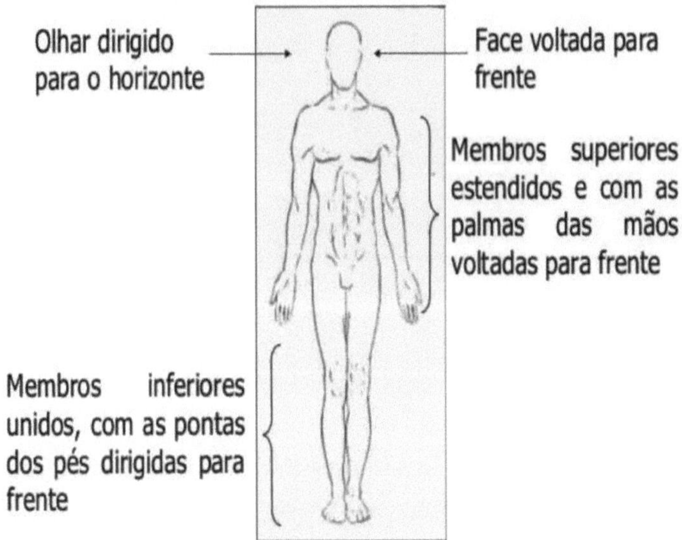

Figure 1 - Anatomical position.
Source: Anatomical Position. Available at:< http://slideplayer.com.br/slide/2908353/>. Accessed on: 13 Jan. 2018.

According to Rizzo (2012, p. 413), as the body metabolises the various foods and nutrients ingested via the digestive tract, the body's cells produce metabolic waste in the form of carbon dioxide, heat and water. The breakdown of proteins into amino acids and the consequent metabolism of amino acids produces nitrogenous waste such as ammonia. Harmful ammonia is transformed into less harmful urea by liver enzymes. The body accumulates excess ions of sodium, chlorine, potassium, hydrogen, sulphate and phosphate.

The function of the urinary system is to maintain the balance between these products and remove excesses from the blood. This system helps keep the body in homeostasis, both by removing and restoring the desired volumes of solute and water from the blood.

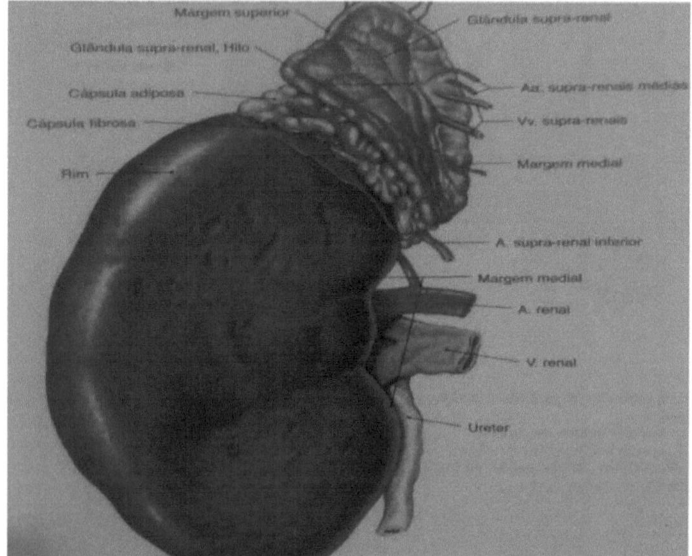

Figure 2 - Anterior view of the kidney

Source: RIZZO,C,D. Fundamentals of Anatomy and Physiology. São Paulo: Cengage Learning, 2012.

For Meldau (2018, p.6):

> The kidneys are paired organs, shaped like a bean, found just above the waist, between the peritoneum and the back wall of the abdomen. It has a brownish-red colour. [a] They are located on each side of the spine, in front of the upper region of the posterior wall of the abdomen, extending between the 11th rib and the transverse process of the 3rd lumbar vertebra. They are described as retroperitoneal organs, as they are positioned behind the peritoneum of the abdominal cavity.

According to Dantas (2018, p. 7), each kidney is about 11.25 cm long, 5 to 7.5 cm wide and a little more than 2.5 cm thick. The left kidney is slightly longer and narrower than the right. The weight of the kidney in adult men varies between 125 and 170g; in adult women, between 115 and 155g. The right kidney normally lies slightly below the left kidney due to the large size of the right lobe of the liver. Above each is the adrenal gland.

According to Magalhães (2017, p. 9), the RENAL HILO (vertical cleft) is located on the medial, concave margin of each kidney, where the renal artery enters and the renal vein and pelvis leave the renal sinus.

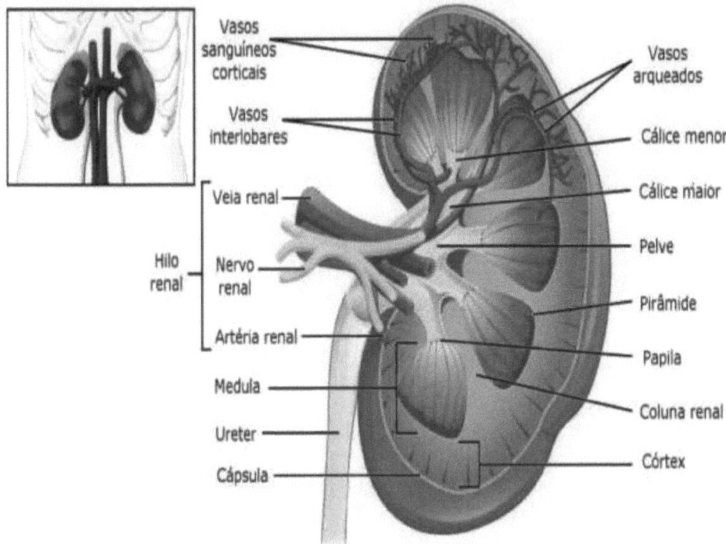

Figure 4 - Renal hilum

Source: Anatomy of the human body. Available at: <http://www.anatomiadocorpo.com/sistema-urinario/rins/>. Accessed on: 5 Feb 2018.

At the hilum, the renal vein is anterior to the renal artery, which is anterior to the renal pelvis. The renal hilum is the entrance to a space inside the kidney. The renal sinus, which is occupied by the renal pelvis, calyces, nerves, blood and lymph vessels and a variable amount of fat. Each kidney has two faces, two edges and two ends. FACES (2) - Anterior and Posterior. Both are smooth, but the anterior is more bulging and the posterior is flatter. BORDERS (2) - Medial (concave) and Lateral (convex). POLES (2) -

Superior (Supra-Renal Gland) and Inferior (L3 level).

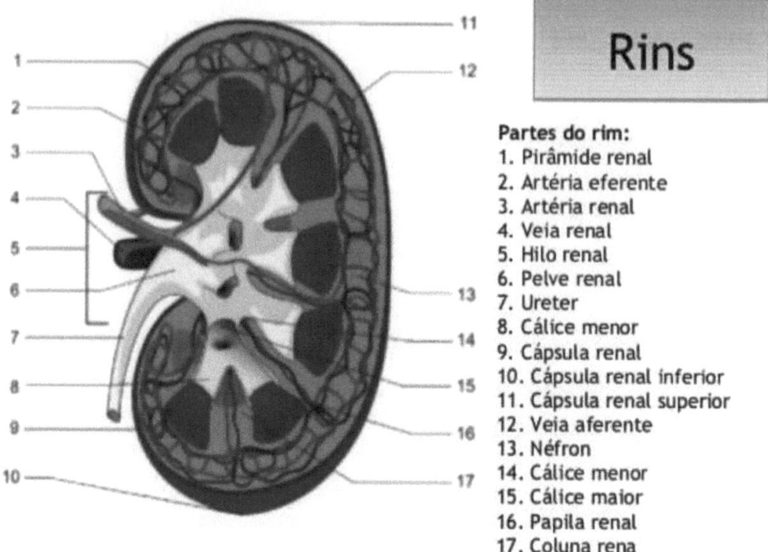

Figura 5 - Internal Anatomy of the Kidneys

Source: Urinary System. Available at:< https://pt.slideshare.net/PedroMiguel156/anatomia- sistema-urinrio-48445792> . Accessed on: 5 February 2018.

According to Rosa; David; Silva (2017, p. 10), the frontal section through which the kidney reveals its external area is called the cortex and an internal area known as the medulla. In a freshly dissected kidney, the cortex is reddish in colour and the medulla is reddish brown.

According to Magalhães (2017, p. 13):

> The medulla consists of 8-18 cuneiform structures, the renal pyramids. The base (widest end) of each pyramid faces the cortex, and its apex (narrowest end), called the renal papilla, points towards the hilum of the kidney. The parts of the renal cortex that extend between the renal pyramids are called renal columns. Together, the renal cortex and pyramids make up the renal parenchyma. Structurally, this parenchyma is made up of millions of microscopic collecting tubules called nephrons, which are functional units of the kidney that regulate blood composition and volume and form urine.

The ducts drain into structures called the minor and major renal calyces. Each kidney has 8-18 minor calyces and 2-3 major calyces. The minor renal calyx receives urine from the papillary ducts of a renal papilla and transports it to a major renal calyx. From the larger renal calyx, the urine drains into the large cavity called the renal pelvis and then out through the ureter into the bladder

urinary tract. The renal hilum expands into a cavity in the kidney called the renal sinus.

1. **2- Anatomy of the Nephrons**

The functional units of the kidney are the nephrons, which are divided into two types: the juxta-medullary nephron, which has Henle's loops that extend into the medulla, and the cortical nephron, which has Henle's loops that do not extend into the medulla. The nephron is basically a microscopic renal tubule, which functions as a filter, and its vascular component (surrounding blood vessels).

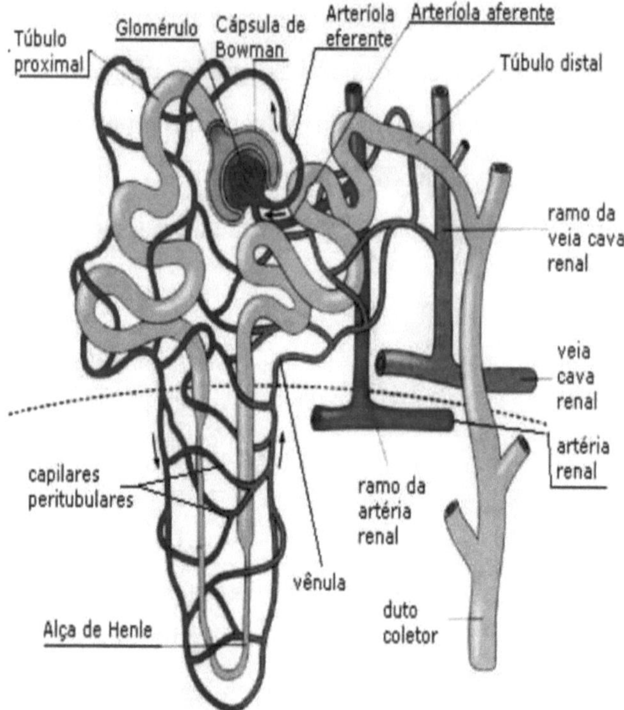

Figura 6 - **Nephrons**

Source: Nephron. Available at:< https://www.infoescola.com/anatomia-humana/nefron/>. Accessed on: 5 February 2018.

For TORTORA, DERRICKSON (2017, p.533), the nephron begins as a double-walled globe known as Bowman's glomerular capsule.

It is located in the cortex of the kidneys. The innermost layer of the capsule is known as the visceral layer and is made up of epithelial cells called podocytes. The visceral layer of podocytes surrounds a network of capillaries known as the glomerulus. The outer wall of Bowman's glomerular capsule is known as the parietal layer.

A collecting space separates the visceral inner layer from the parietal outer layer of the capsule. Together, Bowman's glomerular capsule and the attached glomeruli form what we call the renal corpuscle.

As nephrons are mainly responsible for removing waste from the blood and regulating its electrolytes (which are responsible for the acid or alkaline components of the blood) and liquid content, these structures are richly supplied by blood vessels (RIZZO, 2012, p.416).

The kidneys filter around 1,200 ml of blood per minute. This equates to the blood being filtered approximately 60 times a day.

The kidney's nerve supply comes from the renal plexus of the autonomic nervous system. According to Dantas (2018, p. 23), sympathetic neurons innervate the renal blood vessels by means of noradrenaline. This stimulus causes the arteries to constrict, resulting in a decrease in blood flow and the formation of filtrate. This decreases the formation of urine. The volume of urine production increases in response to the decrease in sympathetic innervation of the renal arteries.

1.3 - Ureters

The body has two ureters, each of which descends from a kidney. The ureter is basically an extension of the kidney's pelvis and advances about 25 to 30 cm downwards until it reaches the bladder (Magalhães, 2017, p. 25). Each one begins as the renal pelvis, in the shape of a funnel, and descends parallel to the spine to the bladder. They then connect to the bladder.

According to Dantas (2018, p. 28):

> The main function of the ureters is to transport urine from the renal pelvis to the urinary bladder. Urine is transported through the ureters mainly by peristaltic contractions of their smooth muscle walls, with gravity and hydrostatic pressure also contributing. Consuming too much liquid causes more urine to be formed per unit of time.

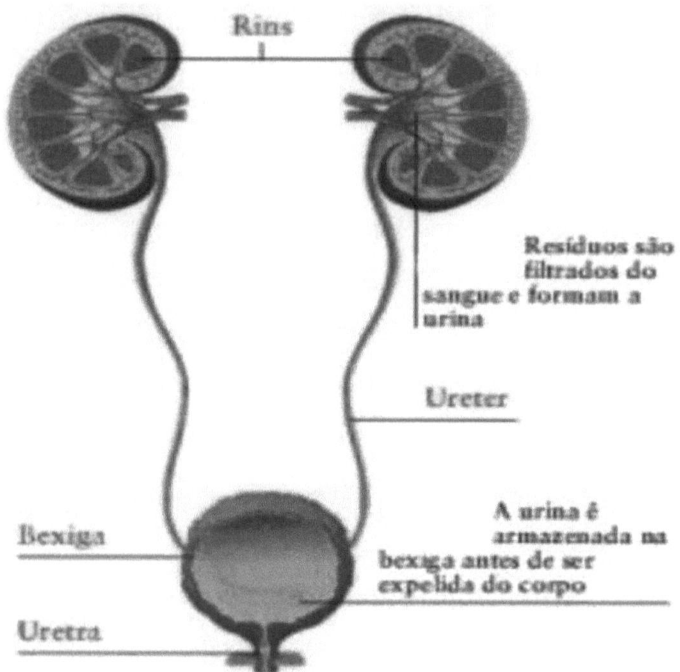

Figura 7 - **Ureters**

Source: Ureters. Available at: < https://www.tuasaude.com/rim-inchado/> . Accessed 9 Feb 2018.

7.4 - Urinary Bladder

The bladder is a hollow muscular organ located in the pelvic cavity posterior to the pubic symphysis. It is made up of the same layers of tissue as the ureters and is a mobile organ held in position by the folds of the peritoneum. When empty, it resembles an empty balloon, when slightly filled with urine, it takes on a spherical shape. As the volume of urine increases, the bladder becomes pear-shaped, occupying more volume in the abdominal cavity. Bladder infections tend to develop in the region of the trigone (Rizzo, 2012, p. 423).

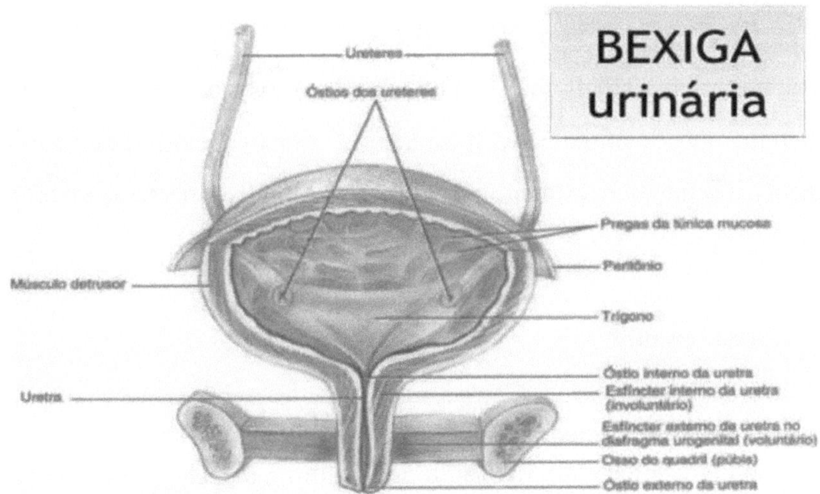

Figura 8 - **Urinary Bladder**

Source: Urinary Bladder. Available at:< https://pt.slideshare.net/PedroMiguel156/anatomia-sistema-urinrio-48445792>. Accessed on: 9 Feb 2018.

According to the Brazilian Society of Anatomy, urine is expelled from the bladder by the action known as urination. This response is caused by a combination of involuntary or voluntary nerve impulses. The bladder has an average capacity of 500 ml. According to Rosa; David; Silva (2017, p. 32), when the volume of urine reaches 200 to 400 ml, the stretch receptors in the bladder wall transmit nerve impulses to the lower part of the spinal cord, which triggers the conscious desire to expel urine and the unconscious reflex called the micturition reflex. During urination, the detrusor muscle of the bladder contracts, as do the muscles of the pelvic floor and abdominal wall. The external urinary sphincter, made up of skeletal muscles that surround the urethra as it exits the bladder, needs to relax in order for the urine to come out and for the bladder to move through the urethra to the outside (TORTORA, DERRICKSON, 2017, p.541).

1.5- Urethra

The urethra is a small, thin-walled tube that runs from the floor of the bladder to the outside of the body. It transports urine by means of peristaltic movements. Its position in men and women is slightly different, as is its function.

1.5.1 -Female urethra

In women, it is located directly posterior to the pubic symphysis and is located on the vaginal wall, in an anterior position, just above the vaginal opening. Its length is around 3.8 cm. It is located between the clitoris and the vaginal opening.

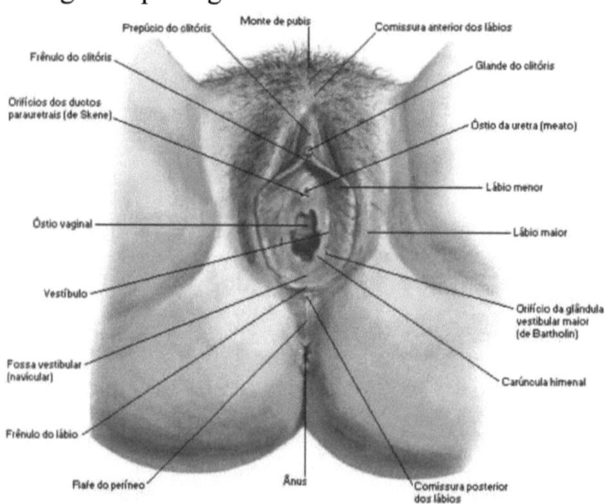

Figura 9 **- Female Urethra**

Source: Female Urethra . Available at :< https://www.auladeanatomia.com/novosite/sistemas/sistema-genital/sistema-genital-female/external organs/>. Accessed on: 9 February 2018.

1.5.2 - Male urethra

The urethra is about 20 cm long and is located directly below the bladder, passing perpendicular to the prostate gland. It then passes through the urogenital diaphragm into the penis and opens into the urethral orifice. In men, the urethra has a dual function: it is part of the urinary and reproductive systems, transporting urine and semen out of the body respectively.

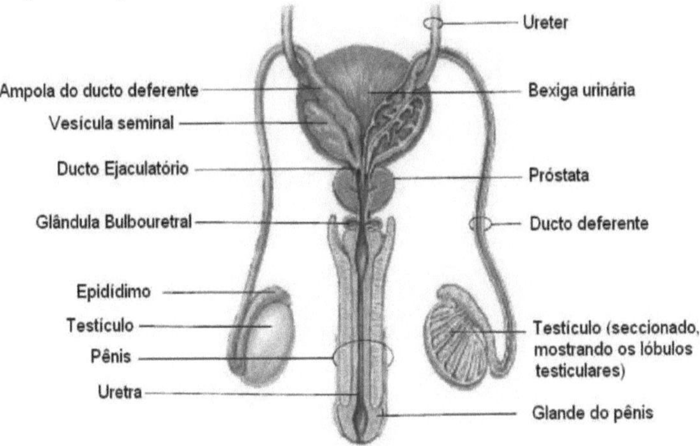

Figura 10 **Male Urethra**

Source: Male Urethra . Available at :< https://sites.google.com/site/planejamentoensinoeservico/fisiologia-do-aparelho- reproductive-anatomy-masculine-1>. Accessed on: 9 February 2018.

Physiology

According to Aries (2008, p. 680), the kidneys are the organs responsible for maintaining the volume and composition of the individual's extracellular fluid within the physiological limits compatible with life.

According to SOUZA; ELIAS (2006, p. 450):

> Urine formation begins in the glomerulus, where 20 % of the plasma that enters the kidney via the renal artery is filtered thanks to the hydrostatic pressure of the blood in the glomerular capillaries. The remaining 80 per cent of plasma, which has not been filtered, circulates along the glomerular capillaries reaching the efferent artery, from where it goes to the peritubular capillary circulation.

The filtrate is a fluid similar in composition to plasma, but with few proteins and macromolecules, since the size of these

substances makes it difficult for them to be filtered through the renal glomerulus wall. Leão (2011, p.6).

According to Aires (2008, p. 677), after its formation, the glomerular filtrate travels through the renal tubules and its composition and volume are then modified by the tubular reabsorption and secretion mechanisms that exist throughout the nephron.

TORTORA; DERRICKSON (2017, p.543), renal tubular reabsorption is the process of transporting a substance from the tubular interior to the blood surrounding the tubule; the mechanism in the opposite direction is called tubular secretion.

The term renal excretion refers to the elimination of the final urine through the urethra.

In addition to glomerular filtration, the renal clearance process can also be carried out by tubular secretion, since the blood that has passed through the glomeruli and has not been filtered passes through a second capillary network, the peritubular one. On the other hand, thanks to tubular reabsorption, many substances after being filtered return to the blood, which passes through the peritubular capillaries and enters the systemic circulation via the renal vein that leaves the organ. (MOREIRA;BARROS, 2000, p. 31).

Dibona (2000, p. 96) reports that the reabsorption and secretion of various solutes through the renal epithelium are carried out by specific mechanisms, passive or active, located in the tubular cell membranes. All transport systems are independent.

2.1- Kidney function

The kidneys do the vital work of the urinary system. The other parts of the system are essentially passageways and temporary storage sites.

According to TORTORA; DERRICKSON (2017, p.528), the kidneys help maintain homeostasis throughout the body by performing the following functions:

> Regulating ion levels in the blood: The kidneys help regulate blood levels of various ions, especially sodium, potassium, calcium, chloride and phosphate.
>
> Regulating blood volume and pressure: The kidneys adjust the volume of blood in the body by returning water to the blood or eliminating water through urine. They help regulate blood pressure by secreting the enzyme renin, which activates the renin-angiotensin-aldosterone system, adjusting blood flow in and out of the kidneys and regulating blood volume.
> Regulation of blood pH: The kidneys help regulate the concentration of H ions in the blood by excreting a variable amount of H in the urine.
> Hormone production: The kidneys produce two hormones. Calcitriol, the active form of vitamin D, helps regulate calcium homeostasis, and erythropoietin stimulates the production of red blood cells.
> Waste Excretion: Some waste products eliminated in the urine are the result of metabolic reactions in the body. Among these substances are ammonia urea, from the deamination of amino acids; bilirubin, from the catabolism of haemoglobin; creatine, from the breakdown of creatine phosphate in muscle fibres; and uric acid, from the catabolism of nucleic acids. Other waste products excreted in the urine are foreign substances from food, such as drugs and environmental toxins (TORTORA; DERRICKSON 2017).

2. 2- Suprarenal glands

Dantas (2018, p. 13) states that the adrenal glands are located between the supero-medial faces of the kidneys and the diaphragm. Each adrenal gland, surrounded by a fibrous capsule and a fat pad, has two parts: the adrenal cortex and medulla, both of which produce different hormones.

For Meldau (2018, p.10), the cortex secretes hormones that are essential for life, while the medullary hormones are not essential for life.

The medulla can be removed without causing life-threatening effects. The adrenal medulla secretes two hormones: epinephrine (adrenaline) and norepinephrine. The cortex secretes steroids.

2. 3- Function of the Nephrons

Nephrons perform several important functions. According to Rizzo (2012, p. 420), they control blood concentration and volume by removing water and solutes; they help regulate blood pH, remove toxic waste from the blood; and stimulate the production of red blood cells in the red bone marrow by producing the hormone called erythropoietin.

2.4- Renal haemodynamics

Knowledge of renal haemodynamics is extremely important for studying the physiology of the kidney, because in this organ there is a close correlation between circulation and tubular function. AIRES (2008, p. 694).

Every minute, around 1,200 ml of blood enters the kidneys, which corresponds to 600 ml of plasma. However, during this period, only 120 ml of plasma is filtered in the glomeruli, i.e. 20 % of the total that enters the kidneys. TORTORA, DERRICKSON, 2017, p.461).

According to BRITO; OLIVEIRA; SILVA (2015, p.31), plasma ultrafiltrate lacks the cellular elements of blood and is essentially protein-free; however, the concentrations of salts and organic molecules are generally similar in plasma and ultrafiltrate liquid. After being filtered, this liquid is intensely reabsorbed from the lumen of the tubules into the peritubular capillary circulation, returning to the systemic circulation.

This means that only 1 to 2 ml of urine per minute remains in the final tubules to be eliminated.

2.5- Peritoneum

The abdominal cavity contains various viscera such as the liver, gallbladder, stomach, duodenum, spleen, pancreas, small intestine, large intestine and appendix. These structures are not free inside the abdomen, but are covered and supported by a membrane called the peritoneum.

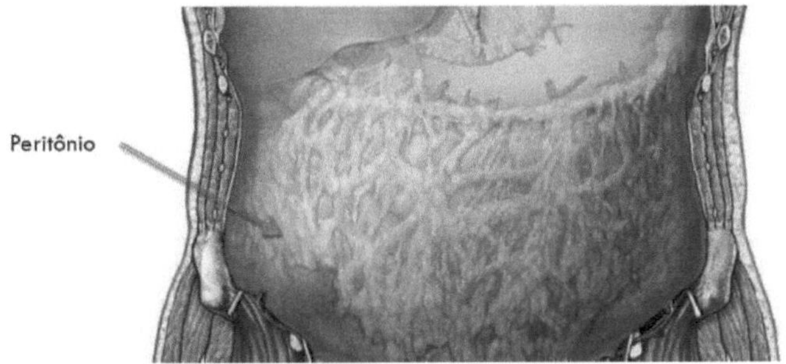

Figure 12 Peritoneum

Source: Peritoneum. Available at:< http://www.anatomiadocorpo.com/sistema-digestorio- apparatus-digestive/stomach/peritoneum/>. Accessed on: 8 Feb 2017.

The peritoneum is divided into two parts: one is known as the parietal peritoneum and completely lines the abdominal cavity; the other, which separates from the abdomen to completely line each of the viscera, is called the visceral peritoneum and makes up around 80 per cent of the total peritoneal membrane. In reality, it is a continuous membrane that covers all the structures.

2.5.1- Peritoneum   folds

After lining each organ, the peritoneum returns to the wall of the abdomen forming a fold that helps to hold the organ in position. According to CARDOSO (2016, p. 6), these leaflets are named according to their shape. They are as follows:

> Epiplon - corresponds to two folds of the peritoneum that join two viscera together. The greater epiplon is an apron-shaped fold from the stomach that joins the large intestine, while the lesser epiplon joins the liver to the stomach.
> Omentum - is the fold of the peritoneum that joins a viscera to the abdominal wall, allowing it to move, as in the case of the mesentery, which joins the back of the abdominal cavity to the small intestine; while the mesocolon does the same, but with the large intestine.
> Ligaments - are extensions of the peritoneum that attach the viscera to the lower part of the diaphragm, especially the liver and stomach.

2.5. 2- Access route for peritoneal dialysis

In cases of renal failure, the kidneys become incapable of performing their filtering function, so it is necessary to carry out a treatment known as dialysis. SODRÉ;COSTA;LIMA (2007, p. 329).

This is a process in which the blood passes through a machine to be filtered and then returned to the circulatory system. SILVA; BRUNE (2007, p. 163).

According to KIRSZTAIN (2007, p. 258), the peritoneum is a membrane that is directly linked to the circulatory system and has the additional property of being semi-permeable, as it allows small molecules to pass through it.

This makes the peritoneum an alternative route for performing dialysis through the modality known as peritoneal dialysis, thus allowing the elimination of waste and excess fluid in the body.

CHAPTER 2

Renal Replacement Therapies

According to the Census of the Brazilian Society of Nephrology, around 12 million people in Brazil have some degree of kidney failure and approximately 95,000 chronic kidney patients depend on dialysis or a kidney transplant to survive.

For SILVA; BEZERRA; SOUZA; et al (2016, p.287), chronic renal failure is related to a decrease in the filtration rate, associated with the loss of the regulatory, endocrine and excretory functions of the kidneys. The forms of treatment for chronic renal failure are: peritoneal dialysis, haemodialysis and kidney transplantation.

1. Peritoneal dialysis

OLIVEIRA; SALGADO; SILVA; et al (2014, p.24), in peritoneal dialysis, we use a "filter" that already exists in our own body. This filter is the peritoneum, a membrane that naturally covers the abdominal organs and also the abdominal wall.

The process is carried out in three stages, according to DAUGIRDAS & BLAKE (2007, p. 23):

> 1. The dialysis solution is placed inside the abdomen.
> 2. While this solution is in the abdominal cavity, impurities from the blood and excess fluids pass through the peritoneal membrane and join the dialysis fluid.
> 3. The liquid is drained and together we remove impurities and excess liquid.

Before starting peritoneal dialysis, a flexible tube called a peritoneal catheter needs to be implanted in the patient's abdomen. This is implanted by a surgeon or nephrologist. Through this catheter, the dialysis solution can be infused and drained. TRISTÃO (2014,p.13).

SILVA; BEZERRA; SOUZA; et al (2016, p.289) describes that the:

> A peritoneal catheter is permanent and does not hurt. It is about 0.6 cm in diameter and 10 to 15 cm long outside the body, usually located 2 cm below and next to the navel. It's flexible and when it's not in use it's fixed to the body with the help of a micropore adhesive plaster and hidden under the patient's clothes. Normally the catheter (which measures around 0.6 cm in diameter) is placed 2 cm below and to the side of the navel. Only 10 to 15 cm remain outside your body. You and your doctor can plan where to place the catheter so that it is comfortable and hidden by clothing.

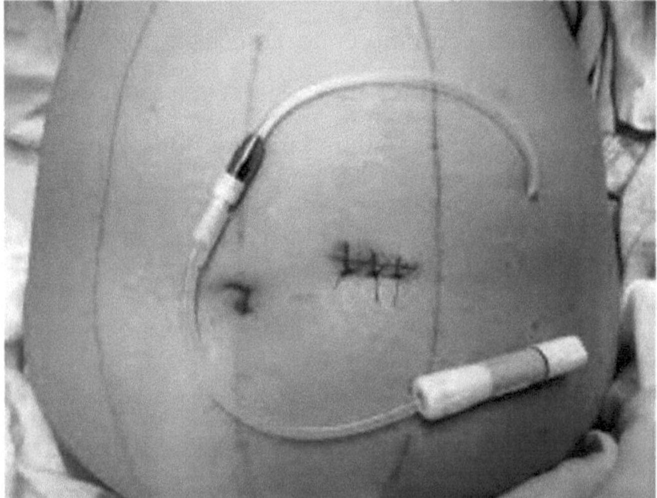

Figure 13 Peritoneal dialysis

Source: Peritoneal Dialysis. Available at: <http://saudeexperts.com.br/dialise-peritoneal/>. Accessed on: 9 February 2018.

BRUNNER & SUDDARTH (2011, p. 1345) state that the goals of peritoneal dialysis are to remove toxins and metabolic degradation products and to restore normal hydroelectrolytic balance.

Peritoneal dialysis can be the treatment of choice for patients with kidney failure who are unable or unwilling to undergo haemodialysis or kidney transplantation.

Sterile dialysate fluid is introduced into the peritoneal cavity via an abdominal catheter at certain intervals.

MORAES (2011, p. 188), the sterile solution is already in the peritoneal cavity and the uremic toxins, such as urea and creatinine, begin to be cleared from the blood.

For DAUGIRDAS & BLAK (2007, p.25):

> Diffusion and osmosis occur as degradation products move from an area of higher concentration (the bloodstream) to an area of lower concentration (the dialysate fluid) through a semi-permeable membrane (the peritoneum). This movement of solute from the blood to the dialysate fluid is called clearance.

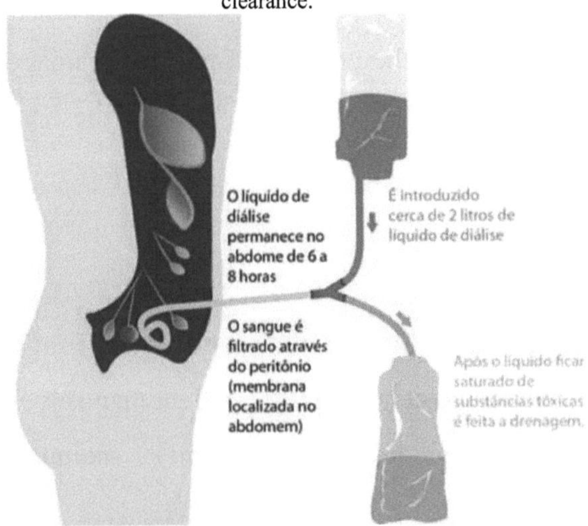

Figure 14 Peritoneal dialysis

Source: Analyses Process , available at : < http://www.ebah.com.br/content/ABAAAfpo0AD/aula-teorica-capd-turma-69>. Accessed on: 9 February 2018.

Ultrafiltration (water removal) takes place in peritoneal dialysis through an osmotic gradient created with the use of a dialysate liquid with a higher concentration of glucose. In general, PD takes 36ª 48h. to achieve what haemodialysis achieves in 6 to 8h.

PD can be carried out using several different approaches: acute intermittent peritoneal dialysis, continuous ambulatory peritoneal dialysis (CAPD) and continuous cyclic peritoneal dialysis (CPPD).

1.1-   Acute Intermittent Peritoneal Dialysis

Indications for acute intermittent PD, a variation of PD, include uremic signs and symptoms (nausea, vomiting, fatigue, altered mental state), water overload, acidosis and hyperpotassaemia. BRUNNER &SUDDARTH (2011, p. 1348).

If the fluid does not drain properly, the nurse can facilitate drainage by turning the patient from side to side or raising the head of the bed. LUGON;MATOS;WARRACK (2010, p.983)

1.2   - Continuous Ambulatory Peritoneal Dialysis

CAPD is the second most common form of dialysis for initial use in patients with ESRD. CAPD is performed at home by the patient themselves or by a trained carer, who is usually a family member. DANTAS;COSTA;VAISBICH (2012, p. 180).

The patient is changed 4 to 5 times a day, 24 hours a day, 7 days a week, at scheduled intervals during the day.

1.3   - Continuous Cyclic Peritoneal Dialysis

The DPCC uses a machine called a cycler to carry out the changes. It is programmed for the amount of liquid to be used and the time required and the number of changes to be made. SAMPAIO; GUEDES (2012, p. 100).

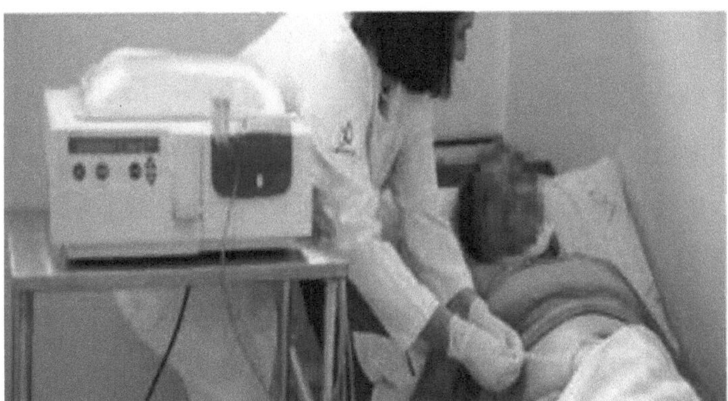

Figure 15 DPCC

Source: DPCC. Available at:< https://www.researchgate.net/profile/Juan_de_Dios_Diaz-Rosales2>. Accessed on: 8 February 2018.

As the DPCC is programmed, it also monitors the course of the total quantities removed and will trigger an alarm if the limits are not met.

fulfilled. It requires one person to set up and dismantle the system (BITTENCOURT; CROSSETTI 2013, p. 243).

CCPD combines intermittent PD during the night with prolonged standing during the day. The peritoneal catheter is attached to a cycler every night, usually before the patient goes to sleep at night.

According to SAMPAIO; GUEDES (2012, p. 97), CPD has a lower infection rate than other forms of PD, since there are fewer opportunities for contamination when changing bags and equipment connections.

It also allows the patient to be free of changes during the day, enabling them to carry out their work and activities of daily living with the greatest freedom.

2. **Acute complications of peritoneal dialysis**

2.1 - Peritonitis

Peritonitis is the most common and serious complication of PD. The first sign of peritonitis is cloudy dialysate drainage fluid. Diffuse abdominal pain and rebound hypersensitivity occur much later. BRUNNER &SUDDARTH (2011, p. 1347).

According to SADALA; BRUZOS; BUCUVIC (2012, p.69), hypotension and other signs of shock can also occur with advanced infection.

2.2 - Overflow

Dialyser leakage through the catheter site can occur immediately after insertion.

> In general, leakage stops spontaneously if dialysis is suspended for several days, giving the tissue surrounding the cuffs located on the abdominal catheter the chance to infiltrate the dacron and close the insertion tunnel. MORAES; PECOITS-FILHO (2010, p. 1035).

2. 3- Bleeding

On certain occasions, a bloody effluent (drainage) can be observed, particularly in young women who menstruate.

The hypertonic fluid pulls blood from the uterus, through the opening in the fallopian tubes and into the peritoneal cavity. Silva ;Bezerra ;Souza; Mendonça; et al. (2016, p.8).

Bleeding is also common during the first changes after insertion of a new catheter, as a certain amount of blood enters the abdominal cavity after insertion. CARVALHO; MAZZALI (2012, p. 88).

2.4- Long-term complications

For BRUNNER &SUDDARTH (2011, p. 1347):

Hypertriglyceridaemia is common in patients who undergo long-term PD, suggesting that the therapy may accelerate atherogenesis. Other complications that can occur with long-term PD consist of abdominal hernias (incisional, inguinal, diaphragmatic and umbilical), probably due to continuously elevated intra-abdominal pressure.

On certain occasions, mechanical problems are observed, which can interfere with the instillation or drainage of dialysate. The formation of clots in the peritoneal catheter and constipation are factors that can contribute to these problems.

2.5- Nursing Care in Peritoneal Dialysis

According to the Brazilian Society of Nephrology, peritoneal dialysis is indicated for patients with acute or chronic renal failure. The indication to start this treatment is made by the nephrologist, who assesses your body through:

- medical consultation, investigating your symptoms and examining your body;

- blood urea and creatinine levels;
- blood potassium levels;
- dosage of acids in the blood;
- amount of urine produced during a day and a night (24-hour urine);
- calculation of the percentage of kidney function (creatinine and urea clearance);
- assessment of anaemia (blood count, iron dosage, iron saturation and ferritin).

The nephrologist and the patient and/or guardian decide by mutual agreement to start treatment. The nursing team must help to clarify and provide the patient with all the information necessary to understand PD, as well as the risks and precautions, this information must be clear and the vocabulary used must be the same as that of the patient. From the outset, the nursing team must also obtain the patient's signed consent, measure vital signs, anthropometric data, record electrolyte dosage values and carry out an abdominal assessment, with the aim of preparing the patient for the procedure.

The main aim of PD is to keep the patient symptom-free and prevent complications of uremia. As we have seen throughout this study, it is essential to correctly adapt this form of renal replacement.

2.5.1 Routine examination and minimum care team.

The dialysis service must periodically carry out the following tests on its patients:

The minimum tests carried out for patients on peritoneal dialysis should be as follows:

a) Monthly: haematocrit, haemoglobin, sodium, potassium, calcium, phosphorus, creatinine and glycaemia for diabetic patients.

b) Quarterly: full blood count, transferrin saturation index, ferritin, alkaline phosphatase, PTH, glycaemia, total protein and fractions and glycosylated haemoglobin for diabetics.

c) Every six months: Vitamin D, total cholesterol and fractions, triglycerides. Perform weekly urea KT/V by measuring serum urea and urea in peritoneal dialysis fluid. For patients with residual renal function, perform creatinine clearance by collecting 24-hour urine and urea clearance by collecting 24-hour urine.

d) Annually: serum aluminium, TSH, T4, PA and lateral chest X-ray, renal and urinary tract ultrasound, electrocardiogram.

e) Possible tests: desferal test in cases of suspected aluminium intoxication; in cases of suspected peritonitis, peritoneal fluid analysis with total and differential leukocyte count, gram bacterioscopy and culture; peritoneal equilibrium test, at the start of treatment and repeated in cases of reduced ultrafiltration and/or inadequate dialysis.

For the peritoneal balance test, it is necessary to carry out a serum creatinine test and two creatinine tests in the peritoneal fluid at different times, and three glucose tests in the peritoneal fluid at different times. Specialised CKD care units should provide patients with antimicrobials for the treatment of peritonitis and infections related to the use of catheters, as long as the patient's clinical conditions allow these infections to be treated on an outpatient basis.

The Continuous Ambulatory Peritoneal Dialysis (CAPD) and/or Automated Peritoneal Dialysis (APD) home programme must include:

a) 01 (one) nephrologist in charge;

b) 01 (one) nurse for every 50 (fifty) patients.

The Hospital Intermittent Peritoneal Dialysis Programme (IPD) must be made up of:

a) 01 (one) nephrologist during the day, to assess patients and attend to any complications, which may be the same as for haemodialysis, DPAC, provided that the ratio of 01 (one) doctor for every 35 (thirty-five) patients is not exceeded;

b) 01 (one) doctor for emergency care at night for every 35 (thirty-five) patients;

c) 01 (one) nurse with at least formal training in dialysis for every 35 (thirty-five) patients during the day;

d) 01 (one) nurse with at least formal training in dialysis for every 35 (thirty-five) patients during the night;

e) 01 (one) nursing assistant on all shifts, for every 02 (two) patients, or for every 04 (four), if all service centres have peritoneal dialysis machines.

3. Haemodialysis

Haemodialysis prevents death, but it does not cure kidney disease or compensate for the loss of the kidneys' endocrine or metabolic activities. DALLÉ (2012, p. 508).

> Haemodialysis is used for patients who are acutely ill and need dialysis in the short term (days to weeks), as well as patients with advanced chronic kidney disease and chronic renal failure DRT who need long-term or permanent renal replacement therapy. LEITE; ARAUJO; LIRA; et al. (2013, p. 5)

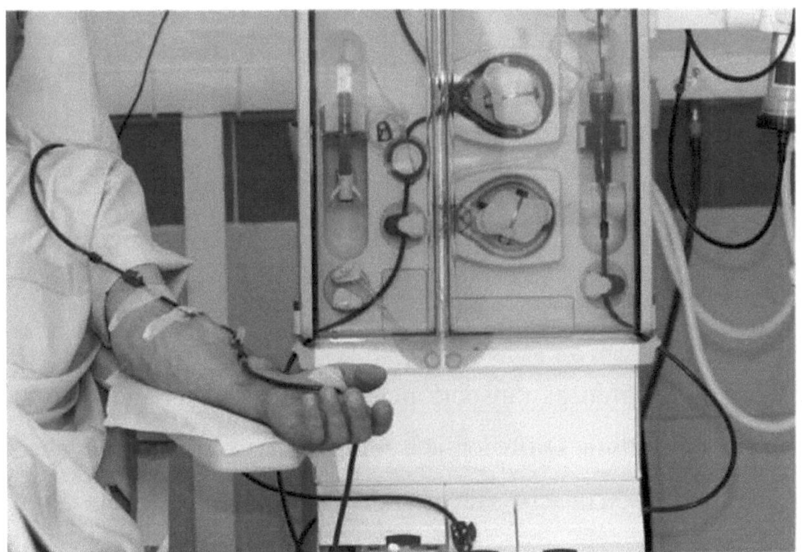

Figure 16 Haemodialysis

Source: Haemodialysis. Available at:< https://www.amato.com.br/content/fistula-arteriovenosa-para-hemodialise-fav>. Accessed on: 9 February 2018.

According to FRAZÃO; MEDEIROS; LIMA; et al. (2014, p. 42), haemodialysis aims to extract toxic nitrogenous substances from the blood and remove excess water.

> In haemodialysis, blood loaded with toxins and nitrogenous degradation products is diverted from the patient to a machine, the dialyser, where the toxins are filtered and removed, and the blood is returned to the patient. Haemodialysis is based on the principles of diffusion, osmosis and ultrafiltration. BRUNNER &SUDDARTH (2011, p. 1339).

4. Kidney Transplant

According to the Ministry of Health's Ordinance 389 of 13 March 2014, every chronic kidney patient has the right to free dialysis or kidney transplant treatment and to receive basic and essential medicines for the treatment of diseases that usually accompany kidney failure.

CHAPTER 3

Peritoneal Membrane Test PET

Peritoneal dialysis (PD), as we saw in the previous chapter, is a method of renal replacement therapy in which the peritoneal membrane allows, by means of diffusion, the exchange of dialytic toxins between uremic plasma and a toxin-free dialysate solution.

There are two peritoneal transport mechanisms for water and solutes: diffusion and ultrafiltration. Diffusion is a solute transport process induced by its concentration gradient across the peritoneal membrane. Ultrafiltration is a solvent transport process induced, in the case of peritoneal dialysis, by the osmotic gradient generated by the high concentration of glucose in the dialysis solution (RIELLA, 2008). In PD, the peritoneal membrane is continuously exposed to a bioincompatible dialysis solution containing high concentrations of glucose, low pH and high osmolarity. The prolonged use of this type of renal replacement can increase the permeability of the peritoneal membrane to small solutes, resulting in inadequate ultrafiltration (FRAZÃO; MEDEIROS; LIMA; et al., 2014).

Another aggravating factor, which is no different from HD, is catheter care. However, when it comes to choosing or needing PD, a study of the patient's socio-economic conditions is needed, as well as an assessment of their self-care, and this assessment should be carried out by the multi-professional team, which will be a key factor in carrying out this renal therapy.

Today, PD is an effective method and equivalent to HD in terms of treatment quality, but it is little used in Brazil. Its use stands out, for example, in some Asian countries and Mexico. In Brazil, treatment began in the 1980s, in Curitiba, by the team of nephrologist Miguel Carlos Riella.

Compared to haemodialysis, PD is a rarely used method in Brazil, according to the 2016 Census of the Brazilian Society of Nephrology, as can be seen in the table below:

1999-2016 DIALYSIS CENSUS. WWW.SBN.ORG.BR

	1999	2016
TOTAL NUMBER OF PATIENTS	42.695	122.825
PD PATIENTS	4.474	9.723
PATIENTS IN HD	38.221	113.122
NUMBER OF DIALYSIS CLINICS	510	757

Source: 2016 Census - Brazilian Society of Nephrology

According to ROMANI - 2015, during the PD process, therefore, a complex and simultaneous variable of phenomena enables the transport of water and solutes. In this process, each patient's peritoneum behaves in an individual way with regard to the transport of solutes and water. Differences in the transport profile of water and solutes have implications both from a clinical point of view and in the prescription of dialysis therapy, making it necessary to classify patients according to what has come to be known as the transport profile of the Peritoneal Membrane - PM.

> To this end, the peritoneal equilibrium test (PET) was introduced in the 1980s. This test was described by Twardowski in 1987 11 and classified the solute transport profile of the patient's MP according to its permeability to medium molecules. It is a method that is still widely used in clinical practice. The test is carried out during a 4-hour PD session with a 2.27% glucose solution in which blood and dialysate samples are taken. The glucose and creatinine concentrations are measured in these samples at 0h, 2h and 4h after infusion of the dialysis fluid (ROMANI, 2015).

Based on the analysis and according to the creatinine ratio between dialysate and plasma (D/P creat) at the specific collection times and the ratio between glucose in samples from different times in the dialysate, 12 collected immediately after infusion and within 2 hours (D/D0 glucose), patients are classified as: high; medium high; medium low and low carriers.

The test is carried out by infusing 2.27% glucose over 4 hours and is based on the balance between plasma and dialysate solutes during this period.

These relationships allow the results to be analysed graphically and transport to be classified as high, medium or low according to the speed of solute transport (Table 2).

Membrane Transport	D/P creatinine (4h)
High	0,82-1,03
Medium - High	0,65-0,81
Medium - Low	0,50 - 0,64
Bass	0,34 - 0,49

Source: ROMANI, 2015 - Traditional pet peritoneal transport classification

According to ROMANI - 2015, the PET-t result's main clinical utility is to serve as a guide for PD prescription. Those patients whose equilibrium is faster Membrane transport D/P creatinine (4h) High 0.82 - 1.03 Medium - High 0.65 - 0.81 Medium - Low 0.50 - 0.64 Low 0.34 - 0.49 22 (high transporters) have an adequate clearance of medium molecules in short spaces of time, However, the rapid absorption of glucose prevents the maintenance of an active osmotic gradient for UF in long stays of dialysate. These patients therefore benefit from the use of automated methods such as automated peritoneal dialysis (APD), in which the time the solution remains in the cavity is shorter (generally around 1.5 hours).

Patients with slow transport (low transporters) need a longer exposure time to the dialysate for adequate clearance of molecules, but the low absorption of glucose allows the gradient to be maintained and ultrafiltration to be carried out for long periods of time; these patients therefore need prescriptions with a longer time for the liquid to remain in the dialysate.

cavity, such as manual infusion methods (DPAC). Inter- and intra-individual transport variability is influenced by age, gender, ethnicity, clinical (comorbidities) and genetic factors, body surface area, solute exposure time and peritonitis. This membrane transport profile appears to be associated with clinical outcomes and survival in PD patients. (ROMANI, 2015).

PET scans are extremely important for defining dialysis prescriptions, as well as helping to analyse problems such as ultrafiltration failure (UF) and to predict more severe peritoneal membrane impairment. The peritoneal transport characteristics for small solutes undergo significant changes during the first month of treatment, becoming stable after this period. Therefore, PET should be performed after four to eight weeks in PD.

CHAPTER 4

Conclusion

Chronic kidney disease (CKD) is a serious public health problem worldwide and is considered an "epidemic" that is growing at an alarming rate. Recent figures indicate that 10 per cent of the adult population has some degree of kidney dysfunction and around 70 per cent are unaware of this diagnosis.

The main risk factors for CKD are diabetes mellitus, hypertension, ageing and family history. Obesity, dyslipidaemia and smoking accelerate the progression of the disease, culminating in the need for Renal Replacement Therapy (RRT). In Brazil, more than 20 per cent of adults have systemic arterial hypertension, 8 per cent have diabetes mellitus, 18 per cent smoke and 50 per cent are overweight.

The most alarming outcomes of CKD are early mortality from cardiovascular disease and progression to end-stage renal disease and the need for RRT.

CHAPTER 5

References

AIRES,M,M. **Physiology**. 3.ed. - Rio de Janeiro: Guanabara Koogan, 2008.

Baroni G. HungaroA. C. Cavalheiro P. Santos K. **Evaluation of the peritoneal balance test in patients undergoing Continuous Ambulatory Peritoneal Dialysis at Santa Casa de Ponta Grossa.** Available at: < rbmi.com.br/artigos/volume2-2015/pg.%2059-67.doc>. Accessed on: 2 February 2018.

BITTENCOURT, G,K.CROSSETTI, M,G. Critical thinking skills in the nursing diagnostic process. **Rev Esc Enferm USP.** 2013; 47(2):341-7.

BLAKE, P. G.; DAUGIRDAS, J. T. **Physiology of Peritoneal Dialysis.** In: DAUGIRDAS, J. T.; BLAKE, P. G.; ING, T. S. Manual of Dialysis. 3ª . Ed. Rio de Janeiro: MEDSI Editora Médica e Científica Ltda., 2003.

BRAZIL. Ministry of Health. **Ordinance No. 389 of 13 March 2014.** Defines the criteria for organising the line of care for people with Chronic Kidney Disease (CKD) and establishes a financial incentive for pre-dialysis outpatient care. Available at: < http://bvsms.saude.gov.br/bvs/saudelegis/gm/2014/prt0389_13_03_2014.html>. Accessed on: 2 February 2018.

BRITO,D,S,I. OLIVEIRA,V,J.**Evaluation of the Bidirectional Relationship between Chronic Kidney Disease and Periodontal Disease in Patients Undergoing Haemodialysis** . Available at :< http://repositorio.saolucas.edu.br:8080/xmlui/bitstream/handle/123456789/2252/ Ingrid%20Silva%20de%20Brito%2C%20Jessica%20Veloso%20Oliveira%20-%20Avalia%C3%A7%C3%A3o%20da%20rela%C3%A7%C3%A3o%20biredici onal%20entre%20a%20doen%C3%A7a%20renal%20cr%C3%B4nica%20e%2 0a%20doen%C3%A7a%20periodontal%20em%20pacientes%20submetid os%2 0%C3%A0%20hemodi%C3%A1lise.pdf?sequence=1&isAllowed=y>.

Accessed on: 15 Feb. 2018.

BRUNNER & SUDDARTH. **Treatise on Medical and Surgical Nursing**. V.1 - Rio de Janeiro: Guanabara Koogan, 2011.
CARVALHO, M.F.C.MAZZALI, M. Glomerulopathies after kidney transplantation. In: BARROS, R.T. et al. **Glomerulopathies**: pathogenesis, clinic and treatment.3. ed. São Paulo: Sarvier, 2012.

Clin J Am Soc Nephrol 10: 1990-2001, 2015 **by *Rajnish Mehrotrae cols from the* Kidney** Research Institute, University of Washington, Seattle, Washington; Department of Medicine, University of California, Irvine, Orange, California; and Department of Medicine, University of Tennessee, Memphis, Tennessee ***entitled:* "Peritoneal Equilibration Test and Patient Outcomes"**.

DALLÉ, J; LUCENA, A,F. Nursing diagnoses identified in hospitalised patients during haemodialysis sessions. **Acta Paul Enferm**. 2012; 25(4):504-10.

DANTAS, O,D,A,H. **Urinary System.** Available at:< http://ulbra-to.morfologia/2011/08/17/Sistema-br/morfologia/2011/08/17/Sistema-Urinario >. Accessed on: 8 Feb.2018.
DANTAS, M.; COSTA, R.S.; VAISBICH, M.H. Glomerulopathy of minimal lesions. In: BARROS, R.T. et al. **Glomerulopathies**: pathogenesis, clinic and treatment. 3. ed. São Paulo: Sarvier, 2012.

DAUGIRDAS, J.T.; BLAKE, P. **Manual of Dialysis**. Rio de Janeiro, RJ: Guanabara Koogan, 2007.

FRAZÃO, C,M. ARAÚJO,A,D. LIRA,A,L. Implementation of the nursing process for patients undergoing haemodialysis. **Rev Enferm UFPE**. 2013; 7(n. esp):824-30.

KIRSZTAJN, M,G. Evaluation of glomerular filtration rate. **J Bras Patol Med** Lab. 2007Aug;43(4):257-64.

LEITE,E,M.ARAÚJO,A,R. LIRA, A,L. SILVA, F,S, OLIVEIRA, A,C, LIMA,C,F. Clinical profile of patients undergoing haemodialysis. **Rev Paraninfo Digital**. 2013; 2(3):1-8.

LEÃO, M,R. **Renal** Physiology: **Filtration and renal haemodynamics and nephron transport**. 5.ed. Bern Fisiologia,2017.

LOBO, J,V,D. VILLAR, K,R. ANDRADE Jr, M,P. BASTOS K,A. Predictors of peritonitis in patients on a peritoneal dialysis programme. **J Bras Nefrol.** 2010. Available at: < http://www.scielo.br/pdf/jbn/v32n2/v32n2a04.pdf>. Accessed on: 2 February 2018.

LUGON, J., MATOS, J.P.S.d. & WARRACK, E.A. Haemodialysis. In: RIELLA, M,C.
Principles of Nephrology and hydroelectrolytic disorders. 5. ed. Rio de Janeiro, RJ: Guanabara Koogan, 2010.1264 p. p.980-1019.

MAGALHÃES, L. **Kidneys.** Available at:< https://www.todamateria.com.br/rins/ >. Accessed on 8 Feb. 2018.

MELDAU, C,D. **Kidney.** Available at: < https://www.infoescola.com/sistema- urinary/kidney/>. Accessed on: 8 February 2018.

MORAES, T.P.D. PECOITS-FILHO, R. Peritoneal dialysis. In: RIELLA, M, C.
Principles of Nephrology and hydroelectrolytic disorders. 5. ed. Rio de Janeiro, RJ: Guanabara Koogan, 2010.

MOREIRA, R,P. BARROS, E. **Update on renal physiology and physiopathology: physiopathological bases of myopathy in chronic renal failure.** J Bras Nefrol. 2000.

OLIVEIRA,A,E,F. SALGADO,C,L. SILVA,G,A,D,S. et al. **Modalities of renal replacement therapy: haemodialysis and peritoneal dialysis.**Carreira Ribeiro (Org.). - São Luís, 2014.

RIZZO,D. **Fundamentals of Anatomy and Physiology.** 3.ed. - São Paulo: Cengage Learning, 2012.

ROMANI, F. Rafael. **Evaluation of the transport characteristics of the peritoneal membrane by comparing three methods (traditional PET, mini-PET and modified PET).** Federal University of Paraná. Available at: https://dspace.c3sl.ufpr.br/bitstream/handle/1884/49048/R%20-%20D%20-%20RAFAEL%20FERNANDES%20ROMANI.pdf?sequence=1&isAllowed=y . Accessed on: 15 Feb. 2018.

SADALA,M,L,A. BRUZOS, G,A,S.PEREIRA, E,R. BUCUVIC, E,M. The lived experience of patients on home peritoneal dialysis: a phenomenological approach. **Rev Lat Am Enfermagem**. 2012; 20(1):68-75.

SAMPAIO C,F.GUEDES,M,V,C. The nursing process as a strategy for developing self-care competences. **Acta Paul Enferm**. 2012; 25(n. esp 2):96-103.

SESSO, R,C. LOPES, A,A. THOMÉ,F,S. LUGON,J,R. et al. **Chronic dialysis in Brazil** - 2011 Brazilian dialysis census report.

SILVA, D,R,A,R.BEZERRA,X,M.SOUZA,N,L,V.MENDONÇA,D,O,E,A.et al. Nursing diagnoses, outcomes and interventions for patients on peritoneal dialysis. **Acta Paul Enferm**. 2016; 29(5):486-93. 4.

Brazilian Society of Anatomy. Available at: <http://www.sbanatomia.org.br/>. Accessed 12 Feb. 2018.

Brazilian Society of Nephrology (SBN). Dialysis census 2013. Available at:< https://sbn.org.br/>. Accessed on: 5 February 2018.

SODRÉ F,L. COSTA J,C,B. Assessment of renal function and injury: a laboratory challenge. **J Bras Patol** Med Lab. vol.43, n.5, 2007 Oct;43(5):329-37. Available at:< http://www.scielo.br/scielo.php?pid=S1676-24442007000500005&script=sci_abstract&tlng=pt>. Accessed on: 15 February 2018.

SOUZA, L,HM. ELIAS,O,D. **Fundamentals of cardiopulmonary bypass.** 2. ed. - São Paulo: Centro editoral. 2006.
SILVA M,M,H. BRUNE, M,F,S,S. Importance of calculating glomerular filtration rate in assessing adult renal function. **Rev Bras Farm**. 2011;92(3):160-5.

SILVA, R,A,R.BEZERRA,X,M.SOUZA,N,L,V. et al Children with kidney disease: association between nursing diagnoses and their components. **Acta Paul Enferm**. 2017; 30(1):73-9. 7.

TEIXEIRA, P. S. RIELLA, M. C. **Protein, carbohydrate and lipid metabolism in renal failure.** In: RIELLA, M. C.; MARTINS, C. Nutrição e o rim. 3ª . Ed. Rio de Janeiro: Ed Guanabara Koogan, 2011.

TORTORA,J,G. DERRICKSON,B. **Human Body: Fundamentals of Anatomy and Physiology.** 10.ed. - Porto Alegre: Artmed, 2017.

43

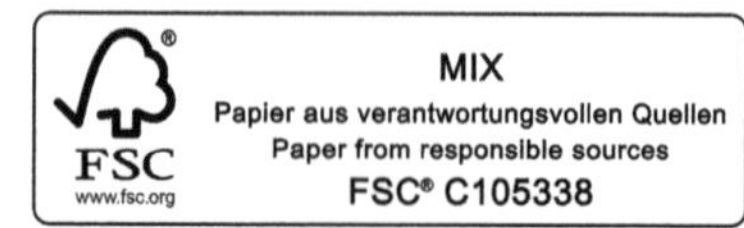

Printed by Books on Demand GmbH, Norderstedt / Germany